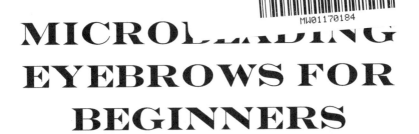

MICROBLADING EYEBROWS FOR BEGINNERS

Ultimate Guide To Techniques For Shaping, Mapping, Pigment Selection, Skin Prep, And Aftercare

DR. KYLE STEFAN

Disclaimer:

The data in this book, is solely meant to be informative and instructional.

This book is not intended to replace expert medical advice, diagnosis, or care. No medical, health, or other professional services are offered by the author, publisher, or any affiliated parties

Individual outcomes may differ in the practice of these therapies, which entail a variety of approaches and methodologies.

A one-on-one session with a trained or certified healthcare professional is still preferable. It is best to consult a trained healthcare provider before making any decisions regarding your health.

The author of this book is not affiliated with any specific website, product, or organization related to any of these therapies.

All reasonable measures have been taken by the author and publisher to guarantee the authenticity and dependability of the material contained in this book.

Table of Contents

ABOUT THIS BOOK

"Microblading Eyebrows for Beginners" serves as an essential guide for anyone entering the world of microblading, offering a complete foundation in the technical, aesthetic, and client-focused aspects of the art. This book emphasizes a deep understanding of eyebrow anatomy, shedding light on the natural structure, growth patterns, and unique variations of brow shapes. Knowing these fundamentals is critical, as they form the basis for crafting personalized, balanced, and flattering brow designs for each client. By exploring the key factors in brow design, the reader is prepared to assess and choose shapes that enhance their client's facial features, giving them a competitive edge in creating high-quality results. The book's insights into the tools and materials used, from microblading blades to pigments suited to various skin tones, equip beginners with the knowledge to make informed choices. A strong focus on hygiene and sanitation practices helps reinforce the book's commitment to professional standards, making it a must-have for new artists who prioritize both aesthetic skill and client safety.

Preparation is a vital element of successful microblading, and this guide covers every detail, from initial consultations to creating a welcoming environment. These preparatory steps build trust with clients, encouraging open discussions about expectations and specific skin considerations. The book guides readers through the importance of pre-procedure care, including patch testing and skin assessments, ensuring clients feel confident and informed. Step-by-step instructions for the microblading process itself demystify the artistry involved, with in-depth techniques on mapping, shaping, and stroke application. The careful detailing of each procedural step allows readers to develop their technique, aiming for results that mimic natural hair strokes and create depth and definition.

Aftercare and healing are often overlooked but critical stages in microblading, and this book provides clear, compassionate guidance on post-procedure care. It equips readers with the knowledge to instruct clients on proper aftercare, including what to expect during the healing process and how to avoid complications. This section highlights the importance of follow-up appointments, where clients' results can be assessed and enhanced for long-lasting beauty. The book also delves into touch-ups and maintenance, with tips on refining and preserving the microbladed brows over time. Readers learn how to assess and conduct touch-ups, ensuring the brows maintain their freshness and precision, while also building a lasting rapport with clients.

One of the standout elements of "Microblading Eyebrows for Beginners" is its commitment to addressing common concerns and troubleshooting potential issues. It covers a wide range of client concerns, from color fading to minor mistakes, providing practical solutions to ensure high-quality results every time. By understanding different skin reactions and mastering corrective techniques, readers can approach each client with confidence, ready to address any challenges. The book also includes a thorough FAQ section, offering clear answers to questions clients commonly ask. Whether it's managing expectations about pain, understanding the longevity of results, or knowing when removal may be an option, these answers equip readers to communicate effectively and professionally.

CHAPTER ONE

THE ANATOMY OF THE EYEBROW

Overview Of Eyebrow Structure And Growth Patterns

Understanding the anatomy of the eyebrow is fundamental to achieving natural and flattering microblading results.

Eyebrows are composed of hair follicles, muscles, skin, and sebaceous glands, which together create the structure and texture of the brow.

Each follicle holds a single hair, with the density and thickness varying between individuals. Eyebrow hairs grow in a unique pattern that follows the contours of the face, forming arches and curves that enhance one's expressions and facial features.

Eyebrow growth patterns are typically broken down into three phases: anagen (growth), catagen (transition), and telogen (resting).

On average, eyebrow hair grows for about two to three months before transitioning to the resting phase, during which it may fall out naturally.

This growth cycle varies from person to person and is influenced by factors such as genetics, health, and age.

Importance Of Understanding Natural Eyebrow Shapes

Natural eyebrow shapes are the foundation of a balanced and harmonious face. The shape, thickness, and arch of a brow can greatly influence one's appearance, making it crucial to understand each client's unique features before beginning a microblading procedure.

For example, a high arch can create a lifted, youthful look, while flatter brows can create a softer, more relaxed expression. Some clients may naturally have fuller, rounded brows, while others have thinner or more angular shapes.

When working with a client, identifying their natural brow shape helps avoid a drastic change that may look artificial. Instead, understanding their original shape allows for subtle enhancement.

By respecting the natural form of the brow, you can achieve results that blend seamlessly with the client's facial structure, highlighting their best features.

Key Factors In Designing The Perfect Brow

Designing the perfect brow requires careful attention to symmetry, proportion, and alignment. Each brow should ideally start from the same point near the bridge of the nose, with the highest point of the arch aligning with the outer edge of the iris when the client looks straight ahead. The end of the brow should extend slightly beyond the outer corner of the eye to balance and frame the face.

It's also essential to consider the thickness of the brow about the client's natural hair density and face shape.

Thicker brows can make a bold statement but may not be suitable for every individual; thinner, more precise lines can be equally attractive if they complement the client's overall look.

To create a polished, symmetrical appearance, measuring tools like calipers or brow mapping pencils are used to ensure each eyebrow mirrors the other as closely as possible.

Common Eyebrow Shapes And Their Features

Different eyebrow shapes can create a range of effects and expressions. Some common eyebrow shapes include:

Rounded Brows: A soft, rounded brow arch creates a friendly and approachable look, ideal for clients with angular face shapes who want to balance their features.

Soft Angled Brows: This shape starts with a soft, low arch and gently rises to a defined peak before tapering off. It adds subtle definition without appearing overly dramatic.

High-Arched Brows: Characterized by a pronounced arch, this shape adds height and can make the eyes appear larger, providing a youthful, lifted effect.

This shape suits those looking to create a bolder, more defined brow.

Flat Brows: With minimal arch and a more horizontal structure, flat brows create a more relaxed, serene expression. These are often chosen by clients with longer face shapes, as they can help reduce the appearance of length.

S-Shaped Brows: This shape has a subtle curve that creates a slight S shape. It works well for clients with unique face shapes or those who prefer a more playful, non-traditional look.

Understanding these common eyebrow shapes and their effects can help in designing a brow style that meets the client's preferences while harmonizing with their facial features.

Tools For Measuring And Assessing Eyebrow Dimensions

Precise measurements are crucial to achieving balanced and proportional eyebrows in microblading. Several tools aid in measuring and assessing the natural brow dimensions:

Calipers: These precision tools measure the distance between various points on the brow and help ensure both symmetry and accuracy. Calipers can measure the brow's start, arch, and endpoints, providing consistency across both brows.

Brow Mapping Pencils and String: Brow mapping pencils are used to mark key points on the client's face to guide the placement of the brows. String is another tool that can be dipped in brow pigment and used to draw lines across the face, aligning the starting point, arch, and tail for a balanced look.

Golden Ratio Compass: Based on the principle of the golden ratio, this compass helps to design a brow shape that aligns with the natural balance of the client's facial features. The golden ratio tool can be particularly helpful when creating brows that are both natural and aesthetically pleasing.

Eyebrow Rulers: Adhesive eyebrow rulers are placed directly onto the client's brow area, providing a quick visual guide for alignment. These rulers are ideal for beginners as they are easy to use and help to establish a consistent baseline.

Using these tools, even those new to microblading can approach the process with precision, creating beautifully balanced brows that enhance each client's natural beauty.

CHAPTER TWO

TOOLS AND MATERIALS NEEDED

Essential Tools For Microblading

Microblading requires several core tools to ensure precision and effectiveness in creating natural-looking eyebrows. Key among these are the microblading pen and blade, which work together to make tiny cuts on the skin where pigment will be deposited.

The microblading pen holds a small, often disposable, blade composed of multiple fine needles, arranged to create hair-like strokes.

Additionally, pigment containers or ink rings are used to hold the chosen pigment close at hand, providing ease of access and reducing the need to dip frequently during the procedure.

Alongside the primary tools, other essentials include numbing creams or gels to make the experience more comfortable for clients, as well as brow mapping tools like calipers and pre-inked string to ensure symmetry. Finally, precision tools like microbrushes help to apply pigments and cleaners delicately, supporting precise application and optimal results.

Overview Of Different Types Of Microblading Blades

Microblading blades come in various sizes and configurations, each suited to different effects and areas of the brow. Straight blades, which are composed of needles aligned in a straight line, are ideal for creating straight, individual strokes that mimic natural eyebrow hairs. On the other hand, slanted or angled blades, where the needles are arranged at an angle, provide easier access to harder-to-reach areas, allowing the artist to maneuver around the brow's natural arch and contours more comfortably.

Curved blades offer a unique advantage for those seeking a softer, feathered look, as they create strokes that curve slightly, blending well with the brow's natural shape. U-shaped blades, recognizable by their "U" formation, are particularly useful for creating strokes with a natural flow in all directions. With these various blade types, an artist can blend different strokes for a more natural, multidimensional appearance tailored to each client's facial structure.

Choosing The Right Pigments For Skin Tones

Selecting the right pigment for a client's skin tone is critical in achieving a natural look and ensuring client satisfaction. Pigments are often categorized as warm, cool, or neutral, and understanding this distinction helps artists choose the best match for different skin undertones. For clients with warm undertones, such as those with olive or golden skin, pigments with a reddish or orange base can enhance and complement their complexion. In contrast, cooler pigments, which contain bluish or ashy tones, are ideal for clients with fair skin or those with cool undertones.

It's essential to keep in mind that pigments may appear darker immediately after application but will fade over time. Therefore, starting with a slightly darker pigment is usually a wise choice to achieve the desired long-term result. Artists should also perform a color test by applying a small amount of pigment on the client's skin to observe how it appears, making adjustments as needed to match their natural brow color or desired shade.

Importance Of Hygiene And Sanitization Tools

Hygiene is non-negotiable in microblading, as both clients' safety and artists' reputations hinge on maintaining a sterile environment. Essential sanitization tools include medical-grade disinfectants, which should be used on all surfaces before and after each session, along with disposable gloves, masks, and aprons to protect both the artist and the client from contamination. Single-use tools, such as disposable microblading blades and pigment rings, should be discarded after each session to eliminate cross-contamination risks.

Beyond these tools, proper waste disposal containers are also necessary for the safe disposal of used blades and other biohazardous materials. Each item that comes in contact with the client's skin must be either single-use or meticulously disinfected before reuse. Keeping the tools clean is essential not only for client safety but also for optimal tool performance, ensuring that each blade remains sharp and effective throughout the procedure.

Setting Up Your Microblading Workspace

Creating a functional and organized workspace is key to an efficient microblading session. A well-arranged workspace reduces setup time, ensures all necessary tools are within reach, and maintains a clean environment for both artist and client comfort. Begin by selecting a sterile area with adequate lighting, as high visibility is crucial for creating precise strokes. Many artists opt for adjustable ring lights or magnifying lamps to ensure every detail is visible.

Lay out essential tools in a logical order. For instance, place blades, pigments, and applicators close to the working area, while hygiene supplies like disinfectants, gloves, and masks should be positioned nearby for easy access.

Ensure that pigment bottles, ink rings, and other items likely to come into contact with the client are set up in advance and covered to maintain cleanliness. Additionally, using a comfortable, adjustable chair for the client and a stool for the artist can improve ergonomics, allowing you to work at the ideal height and angle for detailed, fatigue-free work.

CHAPTER THREE

PREPARATION BEFORE MICROBLADING

Client Consultation And Discussing Expectations

Before the microblading process, a detailed client consultation is essential. This is where the artist and client openly discuss what the client envisions, allowing the artist to understand their style, shape preferences, and color choices.

This initial conversation is more than just a discussion of aesthetics; it helps establish a foundation of trust and sets realistic expectations.

During this time, the artist should encourage the client to share any specific goals they have for their brows, such as achieving fuller or more defined shapes or even correcting asymmetry.

Clarifying these expectations early ensures both the client and artist are aligned, reducing the chance of misunderstandings and ensuring satisfaction with the outcome.

Open communication is key here. Clients should feel free to express any concerns or doubts they may have. Questions like,

"What will the healing process look like?" or "How will the color fade over time?" are common and help reassure the client.

By addressing these questions, the artist demonstrates professionalism and attentiveness, which goes a long way in creating a comfortable experience.

Visual aids, such as before-and-after photos or examples of previous work, are also helpful for clients to see the potential outcomes and better understand the possibilities.

Assessing Skin Types And Conditions

One of the most important steps in the preparation phase is assessing the client's skin type and any skin conditions they may have. Skin type can significantly impact the results of microblading, so artists must be well-versed in recognizing different types.

For example, oily skin often results in faster pigment fading and may require more touch-ups, while dry skin generally holds pigment well, allowing for crisper lines and longer-lasting results.

Knowing these distinctions allows the artist to provide personalized recommendations for each client, helping them achieve the best results possible.

In addition to skin type, other factors such as acne, eczema, or recent cosmetic treatments need to be taken into account, as these can affect the skin's healing ability. Artists should ask clients about their skincare routines and any topical treatments they use, as certain ingredients (like retinoids or acids) can make the skin more sensitive and reactive. Educating clients on how their skin type and condition may influence the final look—and any aftercare adjustments they may need—ensures they are fully prepared for what to expect.

Pre-Procedure Care For Clients (Do's And Don'ts)

To set clients up for the best possible results, there are specific pre-procedure guidelines that must be followed. Clients should avoid certain substances, such as caffeine, alcohol, and blood-thinning medications, at least 24 hours before the procedure.

These substances can increase the likelihood of bleeding, which may affect pigment retention and make the process more challenging for the artist. Refraining from heavy exercise on the day of the appointment is also advised, as sweat can interfere with the pigment application process.

Additionally, clients should avoid sun exposure or tanning for at least a week before the appointment, as this can cause irritation and sensitivity in the skin, making the procedure uncomfortable and potentially compromising results. For similar reasons, they should also avoid any harsh skincare treatments, such as peels or exfoliations, in the days leading up to the appointment. By adhering to these do's and don'ts, clients help create the ideal skin conditions for the procedure, allowing for smooth, even pigment application and minimizing any discomfort during microblading.

Importance Of Patch Testing Pigments

Patch testing pigments is a critical safety step that should never be overlooked. It involves applying a small amount of pigment to a discreet area of the client's skin (typically behind the ear or on the inner wrist) at least 24–48 hours before the procedure to check for allergic reactions. Reactions to pigments can range from mild redness to more serious symptoms, so this step is essential in protecting the client's health and well-being.

Explaining the importance of patch testing to clients can also reassure them of the artist's commitment to their safety. Many clients may not realize that microblading pigments can contain a variety of ingredients, some of which may trigger allergies. If the test shows no adverse reaction, the procedure can move forward with confidence. However, if any reaction does occur, it provides a valuable opportunity to explore alternative pigments or to advise the client on other options for achieving their desired brow look without compromising safety.

Creating A Calming Environment For The Procedure

Creating a soothing environment is just as crucial as the technical aspects of microblading. Clients are often nervous before their procedure, so taking steps to create a calm and welcoming atmosphere can ease their anxiety and make the experience more enjoyable. Soft, ambient lighting, relaxing background music, and comfortable seating all contribute to a positive atmosphere. Clients will appreciate these touches, as they help to reduce stress and create a sense of safety and relaxation.

Beyond the physical setting, the artist's demeanor also plays a role. Using a warm, friendly tone and taking the time to answer any last-minute questions can help the client feel at ease.

Briefing clients on what to expect during each stage of the procedure can further alleviate any apprehension. By focusing on both the emotional and physical comfort of the client, artists can create a holistic experience that goes beyond the microblading process itself, helping clients leave with a positive impression and beautiful brows.

CHAPTER FOUR

THE MICROBLADING PROCEDURE

Microblading is an intricate technique designed to enhance the natural beauty of your eyebrows by creating fine, hair-like strokes. This semi-permanent procedure involves depositing pigment into the skin using a specialized tool, resulting in fuller and more defined brows. Understanding the procedure is crucial for beginners, as it sets the foundation for a successful microblading experience.

Step-By-Step Guide To The Microblading Process

Consultation: The microblading journey begins with a consultation. This is an essential step where the technician discusses the client's desired look, assesses their facial features, and chooses a suitable color for the pigment.

It's important to address any questions or concerns to ensure the client feels comfortable.

Preparation:

Once the client agrees on the design, the technician prepares the area. This involves cleaning the eyebrows and surrounding skin to eliminate any dirt or oils. A topical numbing cream is then applied to minimize discomfort during the procedure.

Mapping the Brows: This is a crucial step where the technician outlines the ideal shape and arch of the eyebrows.

Using a brow pencil, they measure and mark points to ensure symmetry. The client should be involved in this process to approve the shape before moving forward.

Microblading: With the design approved, the actual microblading begins. The technician uses a handheld tool with fine blades to create hair-like strokes in the skin.

Each stroke is carefully placed to mimic natural eyebrow hair, and the technician often dips the tool into the pigment to ensure consistent color.

Pigment Application:

After creating the strokes, the technician applies a pigment solution over the brows to enhance the color and ensure longevity. This process helps the strokes settle into the skin better and provides a more defined look.

Aftercare Instructions:

Once the procedure is complete, the technician provides aftercare instructions. This typically includes avoiding water on the brows for a few days, not picking at scabs, and applying a healing ointment to promote recovery.

Touch-Up:

A touch-up appointment is often scheduled four to six weeks after the initial procedure. This allows the technician to fill in any areas where the pigment may not have been taken properly and to refine the overall look.

Techniques For Mapping And Shaping Eyebrows

Mapping eyebrows accurately is fundamental to achieving a balanced and aesthetically pleasing look. Here are techniques to consider:

Facial Proportions: The golden ratio can be used as a guideline for mapping eyebrows. Divide the face into sections to find the perfect start, arch, and end points of the brow. A common method is to use a pencil or ruler to align with the nostril, pupil, and outer corner of the eye.

Customization: Every client has unique features, so it's vital to customize the mapping process. Consider the client's face shape, eye position, and existing brow hair when determining the ideal shape.

Brow Shape Options: Educate clients on different brow shapes such as arched, straight, or rounded, and how these shapes can enhance their facial features. Collaborate with clients to decide on a shape that reflects their personality and style.

Temporary Marking: Use a brow pencil or a specialized mapping tool to create temporary lines on the client's skin. This allows both the technician and the client to visualize the final shape before committing to the microblading process.

How To Properly Use The Microblading Tool

Mastering the microblading tool is essential for achieving optimal results. Here are key points for proper usage:

Grip and Angle: Hold the microblading tool with a comfortable grip. The angle at which you hold the tool will influence the stroke's depth and direction. A consistent angle helps create uniform strokes.

Blade Pressure: Apply gentle pressure when making strokes. Too much pressure can lead to deeper cuts, while too little may not deposit enough pigment. Practice the right amount of pressure on a practice surface before working on clients.

Stroke Technique: Use a flicking motion to create realistic hair-like strokes. Practice different lengths and angles to mimic the natural flow of eyebrow hair. Varying the pressure slightly can also create different effects.

Blade Maintenance: Keep the blades sharp and clean to ensure the best results. Dull blades can lead to uneven strokes and may cause discomfort for the client. Always use new, sterile blades for each procedure to ensure safety and hygiene.

Importance Of Stroke Techniques For A Natural Look

Achieving a natural look is the hallmark of successful microblading. Here are tips for perfecting stroke techniques:

Direction of Hair Growth: Pay attention to the natural direction of the client's hair growth. Mimicking this direction with your strokes will create a more believable and natural appearance.

Varying Stroke Lengths: Use shorter strokes towards the front of the brow, where hair is typically finer, and longer strokes towards the tail. This technique helps create a more gradual transition and adds realism.

Layering: Layering strokes can enhance depth and dimension. Start with the lighter strokes and gradually build up density where needed. This technique can create a fuller look without appearing too harsh.

Color Variation: Use different shades of pigment within the same brow to simulate the natural variations found in real hair. Subtle color changes can enhance the overall aesthetic and make the brows appear more lifelike.

Tips For Maintaining Client Comfort During The Procedure

Client comfort is paramount during microblading. Here are some strategies to ensure a pleasant experience:

Effective Numbing: Apply a high-quality numbing cream before starting the procedure. Allow sufficient time for the cream to take effect, ensuring minimal discomfort for the client.

Communication: Maintain open communication with the client throughout the process. Explain each step to them and encourage feedback. This helps clients feel more relaxed and involved.

Breaks: Offer breaks if the client feels uncomfortable or anxious. A few moments of rest can help alleviate tension and make the procedure more tolerable.

Calming Environment: Create a soothing atmosphere with soft music, dim lighting, and comfortable seating. A calm environment can significantly enhance the client's overall experience.

By understanding the intricacies of the microblading procedure, beginners can ensure they are well-prepared to provide beautiful, natural-looking brows while prioritizing client comfort and satisfaction.

CHAPTER FIVE

AFTERCARE AND HEALING PROCESS

Proper aftercare is crucial for ensuring the best results from your microblading procedure. Taking care of your eyebrows in the days and weeks following the treatment can significantly impact the healing process and the final look of your brows. Here's a detailed guide to help you navigate the aftercare process with ease.

Detailed Aftercare Instructions For Clients

Following your microblading session, it's essential to adhere to specific aftercare instructions to promote optimal healing. Firstly, avoid wetting your eyebrows for at least 7 to 10 days.

This means no washing your face directly over the brow area or exposing it to steam while showering. When cleansing your face, use a gentle cleanser, and be sure to avoid the eyebrow region.

Secondly, refrain from using any makeup or products on your eyebrows during the healing phase. This includes brow pencils, gels, and any skincare products that may contain harsh chemicals. It's also advisable to avoid sun exposure; if you must be outside, wear a wide-brimmed hat or use an umbrella to shield your brows.

Lastly, avoid picking, scratching, or rubbing the brow area. It's natural to feel some itchiness as your skin heals, but scratching can disrupt the healing process and affect pigment retention. Instead, gently pat the area with a clean, soft cloth if you feel discomfort.

Signs Of Proper Healing And What To Expect

Understanding the healing process can help ease any concerns you might have after your microblading session. Typically, the healing process can be divided into several stages.

Initially, you may notice some redness and swelling around the treated area, which is normal. This should subside within a few hours to a couple of days. After a few days, your brows may start to flake and scab, which is a part of the natural healing process. These scabs may appear darker than the actual color of the brows, but don't worry; as they heal, the color will lighten.

Within about two weeks, your brows should begin to look more natural as the initial darkness fades. By the end of the first month, most clients experience a significant healing transformation, revealing the true color and shape of their brows. Keep an eye out for these signs to ensure your healing process is on track!

Common Side Effects And How To Address Them

While microblading is generally safe, some clients may experience side effects during the healing process.

Common side effects include minor redness, swelling, itchiness, and flaking. These are usually mild and can be managed with proper care.

If you experience persistent redness or swelling beyond the first few days, applying a cold compress can help reduce inflammation. For itchiness, avoid scratching. Instead, consider using a gentle, hypoallergenic moisturizer, as advised by your technician.

Sometimes, clients might notice uneven pigment or patches as the brows heal. This can be addressed during the follow-up appointment, where your artist can make any necessary adjustments to ensure your brows look their best.

Importance Of Follow-Up Appointments

Follow-up appointments are a vital part of the microblading process. They typically occur about 6 to 8 weeks after your initial procedure.

During this session, your artist will evaluate the healing of your brows, address any concerns, and make touch-ups to enhance the shape and color.

These appointments not only ensure that your brows heal correctly but also give you the chance to discuss any side effects you may have experienced. It's important to attend these follow-ups, as they help in achieving your desired look and ensuring the longevity of your microbladed brows.

How To Avoid Complications During The Healing Process

To minimize complications during your healing process, adhere strictly to your aftercare instructions. One of the biggest culprits of complications is moisture.

Keeping your brows dry is crucial, so avoid activities that cause excessive sweating, such as intense workouts or hot yoga, for at least a week post-treatment.

Additionally, be cautious with your skincare routine. Avoid products containing active ingredients like retinol, glycolic acid, or exfoliants around your brows during the healing period, as they can interfere with the pigment.

always maintain a clean environment. Ensure that your hands are washed before touching your face or applying any products, and avoid exposure to dirt or bacteria, which can lead to infections.

By following these guidelines, you can significantly enhance your microblading experience and enjoy beautiful, long-lasting brows.

CHAPTER SIX

COMMON CONCERNS AND TROUBLESHOOTING IN MICROBLADING

Addressing Common Concerns Clients May Have

Many clients approach microblading with a mix of excitement and apprehension. Understanding what to expect and being prepared for potential issues can make the process more enjoyable and rewarding.

Clients often worry about pain levels, healing time, and how natural the results will appear. It's essential to reassure them that while they may feel slight discomfort during the procedure, licensed microblading artists use numbing creams to minimize pain.

Other frequent concerns involve aftercare and maintaining the brows post-procedure. Proper aftercare instructions, like avoiding excessive moisture and sunlight, help clients achieve optimal results. Clients should know that any redness, swelling, or mild tenderness is normal and usually subsides within a few days. By clarifying these concerns upfront, clients will feel more comfortable and better informed about the microblading journey.

Understanding Different Skin Reactions

Different skin types respond to microblading in various ways, and understanding these reactions can be crucial for achieving the best results.

Oily skin, for example, tends to hold pigment differently than dry skin, potentially causing the lines to blur or fade more quickly.

Clients with sensitive or acne-prone skin may experience slightly longer healing times, or, in rare cases, temporary irritation around the brow area.

It's essential to note that individuals with darker or lighter skin tones may experience unique variations in pigment retention and appearance. Educating clients about how their skin type might affect microblading results empowers them to set realistic expectations. In cases where clients experience unusual reactions, like excessive itching or prolonged redness, seeking guidance from a professional can prevent complications.

How To Fix Mistakes Or Uneven Results

Despite the skill and precision involved in microblading, minor imperfections may occasionally occur. Uneven results can be due to the natural asymmetry of a client's facial structure, skin healing inconsistencies, or variations in pigment retention. For minor adjustments, a follow-up session known as a "touch-up" is usually sufficient to correct these issues. This session typically takes place about six to eight weeks after the initial procedure and allows the artist to refine the shape and color, ensuring a more balanced and symmetrical appearance.

If mistakes appear more significant or if a client is unsatisfied with their results, pigment lighting or removal options exist. Laser or saline removal are commonly used methods, depending on the depth and type of pigment used. Although these are safe, they should be handled by trained professionals. Additionally, regular maintenance and adherence to post-procedure care can help reduce the chances of uneven fading or patchiness, supporting a longer-lasting and more even result.

Dealing With Fading And Color Changes Over Time

Fading is a natural part of microblading, as pigments gradually lighten over time. Factors such as sun exposure, skincare products, and individual skin types influence how quickly brows may fade. To help prolong results, it's recommended to limit direct sun exposure and to avoid skincare products containing retinol or acids in the brow area, as these can hasten fading.

Color changes can also occur as pigments settle and the skin heals. Brows may initially appear darker immediately after the procedure, but they will lighten by around 30-50% within the first two weeks. Clients may also notice color shifts, such as a slight ashy or warm undertone, due to the body's response to the pigments. Routine touch-ups, typically every 12-18 months, can restore color and definition to keep brows looking fresh and vibrant.

When To Seek Professional Help For Issues

While most microblading procedures go smoothly, some instances require professional intervention. If clients experience prolonged redness, severe itching, or other signs of an allergic reaction, it's vital to consult a professional as soon as possible.

Issues like pigment migration, where the ink spreads beyond the brow area, also warrant immediate attention from a skilled artist or dermatologist.

If clients feel uncertain about their microblading results or encounter complications, seeking advice from the original artist or another qualified professional is essential. Promptly addressing any concerns not only prevents further issues but ensures a better long-term outcome, allowing clients to enjoy the benefits of beautifully microbladed brows confidently and safely.

CHAPTER SEVEN

TOUCH-UPS AND MAINTENANCE

When And Why Touch-Ups Are Necessary

Touch-ups are an essential part of the microblading process. After your initial appointment, it's typical to schedule a touch-up within 6 to 8 weeks.

This session allows your technician to perfect any areas where the pigment may not have settled properly or where the skin has healed unevenly.

Factors like skin type, lifestyle, and aftercare significantly influence how well the pigment lasts, making touch-ups crucial for achieving the desired look.

Over time, your brows may start to fade due to natural skin cell turnover, exposure to sunlight, and even the products you use. Regular touch-ups—typically every 6 to 12 months—ensure your brows remain vibrant and defined. Without these, your beautifully crafted brows can lose their shape and color, leading to a less polished appearance.

How To Assess The Need For A Touch-Up

Determining when to book a touch-up involves a few key observations. First, assess the color of your brows. If you notice significant fading or any patchiness, it might be time for a touch-up.

Also, consider how well-defined your brow shape is; if the strokes appear blurry or are losing their crispness, a visit to your microblading artist can help restore those sharp lines.

Another important aspect is to monitor any discomfort or irritation. If you experience excessive itching, flaking, or changes in the skin texture around your brows, these could indicate that a touch-up is necessary.

Always communicate with your technician about any concerns during the healing process, as they can offer personalized advice on the timing of your next appointment.

Techniques For Refining And Enhancing Brows

During a touch-up appointment, several techniques can be employed to refine and enhance your brows. Your artist may start by assessing the original shape and color of your brows to determine what adjustments are needed. They can use a small blade to add more strokes, filling in any sparse areas and creating a more natural appearance.

Color correction is another technique that may be necessary, especially if the initial shade has faded or changed after healing. Your technician can introduce a different pigment to bring back your desired hue. They might also adjust the shape of your brows to better suit your facial features, ensuring that they enhance your overall appearance. With these techniques, touch-ups provide an opportunity for continuous improvement and customization of your brows.

Client Maintenance Tips For Long-Lasting Results

To maintain your microbladed brows and prolong their results, follow these simple yet effective tips. First, avoid excessive sun exposure; UV rays can fade the pigment more quickly.

When spending time outdoors, consider wearing a wide-brimmed hat or using a high-SPF sunscreen on your brows. This step is crucial, especially in the weeks following your procedure.

Hydration is key for your skin, so be sure to drink plenty of water and keep your skin moisturized. However, be cautious with topical products; avoid oils or creams directly on the brow area that can cause the pigment to lift prematurely.

Additionally, be mindful of the makeup you use. Heavy makeup application over the brows can also affect their longevity. Opt for light powders or avoid brow products altogether. Finally, practice good skin care routines that involve gentle cleansing and exfoliating, but keep in mind that harsh scrubs should be avoided around the brow area to maintain the integrity of the pigment.

Best Practices For Scheduling Follow-Ups

Scheduling follow-up appointments is vital for maintaining your microbladed brows. A good rule of thumb is to plan for your first touch-up 6 to 8 weeks post-procedure, as this is when most adjustments will be made.

After the initial touch-up, you can typically schedule annual touch-ups or sooner if you notice significant fading or changes in your brows.

Consider maintaining a calendar or reminder system to track your appointments. This practice helps ensure you stay on top of your brow care routine without letting too much time pass between sessions. When booking your appointments, communicate with your technician about your lifestyle and how frequently you wish to maintain your brows; they can help tailor a schedule that works best for you.

Remember, every individual's skin heals differently, and factors like your environment, skincare routine, and general health can all play a role in how quickly your brows fade. Adjust your follow-up schedule accordingly and consult your artist for personalized recommendations based on your unique brow needs.

CHAPTER EIGHT

FREQUENTLY ASKED QUESTIONS (FAQS)

What Is The Average Duration Of Microblading Results?

Microblading is a semi-permanent makeup technique designed to enhance the appearance of your eyebrows. The results of microblading can last anywhere from 1 to 3 years, but this duration varies based on several factors, including skin type, lifestyle, and aftercare.

For those with oily skin, the pigment may fade more quickly due to natural oil production, which can cause the ink to break down faster. In contrast, individuals with dry skin might enjoy longer-lasting results as their skin retains the pigment better. Additionally, factors like sun exposure, skincare products, and whether you frequently undergo exfoliation treatments can influence how long the microblading lasts.

To maintain the desired look, many people opt for touch-up sessions every 6 to 12 months. This helps to refresh the pigment and ensure that the eyebrows look their best over time.

How Painful Is The Microblading Procedure?

Pain perception varies from person to person, but many people report that the microblading procedure is relatively tolerable. Before the actual microblading begins, a topical numbing cream is applied to the eyebrow area. This cream helps to minimize any discomfort during the procedure.

Some clients describe the sensation as similar to light scratching or a slight stinging feeling, while others might not feel much at all. The procedure itself typically lasts about 2 to 3 hours, including the design and numbing stages, so it's crucial to stay relaxed throughout the process.

If you are particularly sensitive to pain, communicate this to your microblading artist. They can adjust the numbing technique or provide additional numbing solutions to ensure you are comfortable throughout the procedure.

Can Microblading Be Done On All Skin Types?

Microblading is suitable for various skin types, but specific considerations must be made depending on your skin's characteristics. For instance, individuals with oily skin may face challenges, as excess oil can affect the longevity and appearance of the pigment. Artists may recommend different techniques, such as a powder brow or ombre shading, to achieve the best results for oily skin.

For those with dry or sensitive skin, microblading can yield excellent results, but extra caution should be taken to avoid irritation. It's vital to have a thorough consultation with your artist to discuss your skin type and any concerns.

Moreover, individuals with skin conditions like eczema, psoriasis, or dermatitis in the brow area should consult a dermatologist before proceeding with microblading. Each skin type requires a tailored approach to ensure that the procedure is safe and effective.

How Do I Choose The Right Microblading Artist?

Choosing the right microblading artist is crucial for achieving beautiful and natural-looking brows. Start by researching local artists and reviewing their portfolios. Look for before-and-after photos that showcase their work, paying close attention to the styles and techniques they use.

Next, check for certifications and licenses. A qualified microblading artist should have completed a recognized training program and possess the necessary licenses to practice in your area. Don't hesitate to ask about their experience and the number of procedures they've performed.

Scheduling a consultation can also be beneficial. This allows you to meet the artist, discuss your brow goals, and gauge their professionalism and communication style. A good artist will listen to your preferences, provide insights, and suggest a design that complements your facial features. Trust your instincts; you should feel comfortable and confident in your skills before proceeding.

What Happens If I Want To Remove Or Change My Microblading?

While microblading is designed to be semi-permanent, you might find yourself wanting to remove or change the design for various reasons. If you're unhappy with the results or want a new style, there are a few options available.

The most common method for removing microblading is through saline removal. This technique involves using a saline solution to draw out the pigment from the skin. Multiple sessions may be required, and it's essential to have this done by a skilled professional to minimize skin trauma.

If you're considering a change rather than complete removal, your artist can help adjust the shape or color through a touch-up session. It's important to communicate your desires clearly, as a skilled artist can often alter existing microblading to better match your new preferences.

Remember that patience is key when it comes to microblading adjustments or removals, as the skin needs time to heal between procedures. Always consult with your microblading artist to discuss the best course of action tailored to your specific needs.

Made in United States
Troutdale, OR
01/25/2025

28297582R00037